Lessons From the Cave
The Primal Home

A Guide to Primal Feng Shui
by Renae Jensen

Printed in the United States of America

Kora Press ® is a federally registered trademark.

ISBN *978-0-9912430-0-6*

Published by Kora Press ®
www.KoraPress.com

KO
RA

K O R A
P R E S S

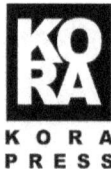

Table of Contents

Dedication
Foreword
Gratitude
Introduction
Beginning
Lesson 1: The Three Laws
Lesson 2: The Tao
Lesson 3: Location, Location, Location
Lesson 4: Fangs, Points and Blades
Lesson 5: Danger from Above
Lesson 6: Invading Energies—
Openings and Doorways
Lesson 7: Evil Lurks in the Corners—
Dark and Hidden Areas
Lesson 8: Meandering Chi—Room Flow
Lesson 9: Color my World
Lesson 10: Gather with Me—
Kitchens and Dining Rooms
Lesson 11: Unity and Connection—Living Rooms
Lesson 12: Our Nest—Bedooms
Lesson 13: Your Living Home—
Spirit, Symbols, Signs
Lesson 14: Space Clearing
House as a Circle of Life
About the Author

Dedication

This book is dedicated to those of you that have a book deep inside of you, waiting to emerge. I encourage you to express yourself. You have wisdom and value that the world is waiting to hear. *Lessons From the Cave—the Primal Home* is my first official book. It has manifested from my experiences, thoughts, and dreams. Pages of notes and stacks of yellow legal pads are finally brought into reality. I am excited and compelled to share the insights I learned through hundreds of consultations, classes, and contemplation.

This book is dedicated to my beautiful daughter Heather and my brother Louis. Their belief in me has given me the gift of trust and faith. I am grateful for the many years they have listened to my faith in man's ability to create peace and harmony—in themselves, their homes, and on the planet.

I hope you enjoy this book and learn to create your sacred space from the innate wisdom that resides deep within you.

Blessings
Renae Jensen

FOREWORD

Unlock the ancient secrets of balance, harmony, and well-being with *Lessons from the Cave: Primal Psychology Feng Shui* by Renae Jensen. As a distinguished Feng Shui master and seasoned educator, Renae brings decades of expertise to illuminate the profound connection between our surroundings and our innermost selves. Embark on a transformative journey as you uncover the primal instincts that shape our interactions with the spaces we inhabit.

In a world that moves at an ever-increasing pace, *Lessons from the Cave* stands as a guiding light for those who seek sanctuary amid the chaos. Renae Jensen masterfully explores the fundamental principles that have shaped human psychology since time immemorial. With clarity and depth, she reveals the profound reasons behind Feng Shui's effectiveness, demystifying its practices and offering pragmatic, easy-to-follow instructions.

Lessons from the Cave reveals the primal psychology principles that resonate within each of us, providing insight into the profound ways our environment influences our sense of security, wellness, and inner equilibrium. Renae Jensen's compassionate guidance empowers you to create living spaces that resonate with your unique essence, fostering a sense of connection with the world around you and supporting your goals.

Paige Saucyn

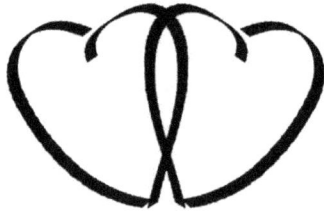

GRATITUDE

With the deepest gratitude to my husband Chris, who has taught me that all things are possible. My children John, Christian, Heather and Corey are my foundation and I want to thank them for all their support. My grandchildren Eric and Anna are the light of the future, and I am blessed to be their Nae-Nae.

With gratitude to my friend, feng shui sister, and angel Lois Kramer Perez for her transformational guidance.

With gratitude to a dear friend Christine Altamuro who always supported the author that was buried deep inside me.

I would like to express my deepest gratitude to my dear student, friend, and mentor Paige. Her wisdom and generosity have been food for my soul. She has been an integral part of sharing the wisdom of Feng Shui and Conscious Design with me. She is a lighthouse for the future.

Introduction

For over twenty years I have been teaching and consulting about the value of creating healthy harmonious homes. I am considered a Feng Shui Master, a title that speaks to my many years of training, teaching, and actively consulting in the field. I "see" the title Master to be an obligation and a responsibility to myself and others. I know of the incredible transformational shifts that are available to everyone.

Today, I see a large surge of interest in Feng Shui and Space Clearing, especially in the industries of real estate and health. I am an active New Jersey real estate agent and have the opportunity to be in hundreds of homes for both buyers and sellers. Many people come to me with interest, questions, and excitement. There is a desire to learn more about Feng Shui. There is also a large amount of confusion, hesitation and overwhelm with the massive amount of information on the topic.

This is a simple book. There are no protocols, fancy practices, formulas, design theories. Everything we need to know, we have been born with. It is innate in our nature. It is deep within us.

Lessons from the Cave reaffirms the importance of bringing our homes and spaces to a place of balance and flow. Feng Shui, called the ancient art of placement, is invaluable to us. We are not only connected to our homes; our homes are an expression of our lives. We spend thousands of dollars healing our bodies and our minds, and we return to sick, unbalanced homes. Let your home be your healing place, a support system that offers a true foundation for your success!

How do you proceed? How do you know what to do? We already have much of this knowledge deep within us. We already know how it feels to be in a safe sound place, and we know when we feel disconnected and stressed. I created *Lessons from the Cave* to remind us of our deep innate wisdom. This book reminds us of our natural state of being. When we apply primal principles

Introduction

to our homes, we create a safe, secure, stable environment that allows us to feel connected, alive, and balanced. This book is not about "learning." It is about tuning into the messages of our internal navigator, our primal brain and instincts.

Renae

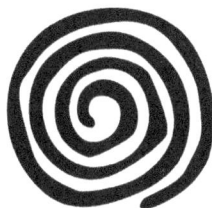

Beginning

There is an overall understanding today that we as a "whole Earth" have reached an impasse. As a modern human family, we are overwhelmed with stress, anxiety and depression. We acknowledge the need to create a massive transformational shift and to find harmony and balance at all levels. Creating safe healthy homes is our first step. Healing one home at a time will begin a ripple that will move into the world.

Personal Survival

Man is washed up on a desert island. His number one instinct is to seek shelter, and then food. Shelter protects us from the elements, wild animals, the weather, and outsiders. A roof overhead, and a door that closes offer security and protection.

Your home needs to be your support system. Creating a feeling of safety and security allows the body to relax and enter the "blue zone" and out of the "flight and fight" response. This can be achieved when the brain and primal instincts are not getting signals of stress and danger. We often dismiss fears and emotions, but we cannot override primal instincts for long without a high cost. Keeping the body on alert 24 hours a day has a high cost—cortisol levels soar, sleep is disturbed, and stress runs the show.

Humans share core fundamentals, even though no two humans are alike. Before we design, renovate, or expand a home design, we need to satisfy the basic human need of "safety and security." As we work to expand our minds, and strengthen our bodies, we often ignore the impact our home has on us. We go home to "sick homes," and our homes become a drain rather than a support system. There are core basics to being human that are the building blocks, and core requirements, that are necessary in our structures to offer us optimal health and life opportunity and experience.

As humans, we are born with five senses, an amazing body and an innate instinct that has allowed us to survive through the centuries. Our primal instincts are just as valuable today as they were thousands of years ago. We have brilliant minds, and our minds can often override our primal intuition and messages. When we disconnect from all the gifts we were born with, we can become robotic, an example of artificial intelligence. The mind can be very methodical, and it can also be trained and manipulated. What are not trainable are our natural instincts, our primal instincts—the ability to see, feel, hear, touch, taste, beyond what the mind can often access.

What is Primal?

When we use the word *primal,* we are referring to a time on Earth when human life was early and primitive. Early man lived intimately with nature and relied on his primal instincts for survival. Early primal basics follow simple rules, imposed by the desire to thrive. When under danger and stress, the body's stress response system and cortisol are activated. The result is what is called a *fight or flight response.* This is considered the evolutionary prehistoric response that allowed the first humans to survive.

The key primal need is that of safety and security—to be safe and sound. My daughter was on a business trip with an impending tornado. I asked her to let me know when she was "safe and sound." What does safe and sound mean? Safe relates to our physical safety and the word sound adds a deeper meaning. Safe and sound is an ancient term that means to be "whole" in body and mind, and free from injury,

Our Homes

Our homes are physical living affirmations to the type of life we are living. The messages we set in our homes will mirror back into our lives as well as resonating out into the universe. Our homes are our second skin—another layer—which allows us another path within which to set our intentions for our lives, our partners and our families.

Even nomadic tribes use distinct, individualized portable housing, tipis, and organized arrangements to keep their homes the same, just moving location to location.

Being homeless deprives the human of his deepest needs. Often the homeless will find a bench, street, corner, or one regular location to call home.

Creating a home that supports and encourages you and your family and learning how to read your homes—what are you really saying to the world, how do you really feel about yourself?

"Whoever invented the house invented more than a building—it was an expression of culture that was shaped by the way people lived, and it shaped our lives in turn. They're more than just the walls around us, or the roof over our heads. Houses teach us about what people believe, who they are, and even what their health is like. Houses are, as Moore put it, "part of the consultable record of what it means to be human."

https://fivethirtyeight.com/features/who-built-the-first-house-and-what-even-is-a-house/

Trusting Your Gut

Humans have a primitive brain that is located in the stomach or "gut" of the body. Called the *Dan Tien* in Chinese medicine practices, this brain is the core and center of our primitive survival mechanisms.

"One of the major functions of the primal brain is to help us distinguish between threatening and non-threatening stimuli."

Beginning

https://www.interaction-design.org/literature/article/our-three-brains-the-reptilian-brain

Today's world may not have the same daily dangers as those that faced primitive humans on a daily basis, but we are still in a world with many dangers, violence and threating situations. Our primal brain has not abandoned us; it is still working to keep us safe and sound. Anything unfamiliar or historically threatening will activate our primal brain. We are either ignoring these alerts, or are numb to their heedings. The result of dismissing our gut alerts is connected to a variety of digestive concerns.

"If you've ever *gone with your gut* to make a decision or felt *butterflies in your stomach* when nervous, you're likely getting signals from an unexpected source: your second brain."

John Hopkins

https://www.hopkinsmedicine.org/health/wellness-and-prevention/the-brain-gut-connection

The goal of *Lessons From the Cave* is to reawaken your connection to your primal instincts and to learn how to make positive adjustments to your home space. It is the most ancient and basic form of Feng Shui known to man.

Lesson One

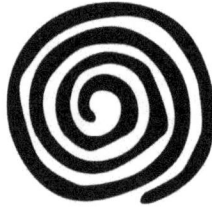

LESSON ONE: THE THREE LAWS

To understand primal Feng Shui, we must first explore the three foundational laws which describe the expressions of all life on Earth; they describe the language of nature. Understood and taught in Chinese medicine and Feng Shui, these three laws bring us to a deep understanding of our connection to ourselves, other people, our homes, and the Earth.

Modern science now offers evidence of the three laws through studies of epigenetics and quantum physics. The study of epigenetics reflects on the development of instincts and the environment's effect on the way genes are expressed. There is a field of quantum physics called Tao science that connects the science of quantum research with the wisdom of the Tao's concept of unity.

The Three Laws:
Everything is connected—Tao
Everything is Alive with Energy—Chi
Everything changes—Yin/Yang

Law 1: The Tao—*Everything is connected*—is the foundation of Feng Shui. We are connected to our space, and our space influences us every day. This is the wisdom of "One." Many ancient cultures understood the power of the relationship between man and his environment.

Do your office spaces, homes, and environments have an effect on you? How much time do you spend in your office, at your desk? Within 30 seconds after entering a space or a room, we begin to analyze and access that room. If we are in a negative room and do not have to spend a lot of time there, the space will not have a lasting impact on us. The longer we are in a space, the more influence the space will have on us, our moods, vitality and health. After three months of being in the same space, you are enmeshed and adjusted into that space on a vibrational level, either positively or negatively.

Law 2: *Everything is Alive with Energy and Life Force*
Chi is the center of all living cells, and this energy creates matter. It is the invisible energy that moves and generates all of life. Yoga, Breathwork, and Martial Arts all develop, enhance, maintain, and control the chi in our bodies. Our environments, homes, possessions, and objects all are alive with energy. To have a healthy home, we need to learn to find, address, and adjust negative energy.

Chi moves in a straight line and in a long straight pathway; it becomes very fast moving. Too much chi is like too much wind and water—causing destruction and damage. Too little chi causes us to stagnate, get sick, and die. Chi can be negative, created by pent up energy and energy that is moving too fast, or by energy that is moving too slow or is stuck.

Here are some types of challenging Chi:

Pent up Chi—creates a feeling of pressure, stress, and explosive anger. It can be experienced in overcrowded trains, planes, or elevators. Too much energy accumulates with no exit of release.

Stuck Chi—creates a feeling of depression or unexpressed anger. An example of stuck chi is to experience a room that has too much furniture or clutter. Movement is challenged and blocked. We feel constrained and angry.

Poison Arrows—a poison arrow is a term used to describe very "pointy" energy that comes towards us that we experience as a threat. Negative chi can be formed by too much acceleration along straight lines, like a speeding bullet. A busy highway has chi, moving in a straight line. This type of road is good for fast

15

travel but tends to make cars crowd each other as everyone seeks to move faster and faster, until you feel as if you are being attacked from behind. Secret or poison arrows aimed at us in the form of roads, other buildings, houses, and objects make us feel vulnerable and threatened.

Law 3: *Everything Changes—Yin/Yang Creating Balance*
We all know the popular Yin Yang symbol: it represents heaven and Earth harmony—the principle of two cosmic forces of the universe. This balanced whole is considered the TAO or the Way. It shows the inevitable and constant motion of life's cycles. This is the principle of dualism: opposites whose existence depends on each other. Opposites that support each other—one cannot exist without the other. Without dark, light cannot exist. Without hot, there is no cold. Without death, there is no life.

In Feng Shui, applying the balance and flow of yin and yang brings good fortune. Bringing balance into our busy lives today is a challenge, but one that we must begin to attempt to realize. A space design needs to incorporate the overall flow of energy, and pace of the purpose of the structure. Each space, whether it is a home, school, hospital or office, will have areas that generate more quiet or yin, or more activity or yang.

Yang spaces create activity, interaction, and communication, and make us want to jump into action. Yin spaces encourage thinking, reflection, and rest. These foundational concepts will be expressed throughout the rest of the book and are the basis for an instinctual feeling of safety.

Lesson Two

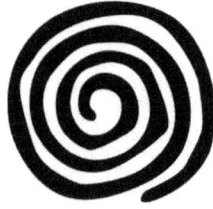

LESSON TWO: THE TAO
Return to Nature

We often feel that we are *in* nature, when the reality is we are nature! Many of us spend little time in nature today. We get in our cars in our garages, drive out the driveways, and our bare feet almost never touch the Earth.

Our disconnect from nature and natural cycles and principles has created many of the huge problems we face today, not only in building materials, but in neighborhood planning, building shapes and designs, and interior planning.

Reconnecting to our core essence in these times is essential to maintain balance. Bring natural elements into your home space. Check your home to see where you can remove unhealthy materials and replace them with green natural products.

Bring in lots of natural light with windows and natural light bulbs. Connect to the natural timing of daylight and nighttime. In the evening, utilize shades and window coverings that allow the quiet of night to soothe us into a deep, undisturbed sleep.

Always create window treatments that allow full control over light and dark. When you are in control of your environment rather than the environment controlling you, you feel empowered and secure. Primal man worked with the flow of nature, understanding how to best situate himself for optimal opportunity and survival.

The Five Elements:
Everything in our living world is created as one of the five ele-

ments The five elements are the language of life, embodying the transformations of all materials on Earth, as expressed in their natural form. The five elements are practiced in many eastern sciences, including Chinese medicine, Tai Chi, and astrology. In Feng Shui, the five elements are used to analyze, adjust and balance the exterior and interior factors of a space.

A balanced home will have each element represented, placed in specific locations to create optimal harmony. We are going to look at how each element affects our physiology and psychology, and how they can be expressed in a room.

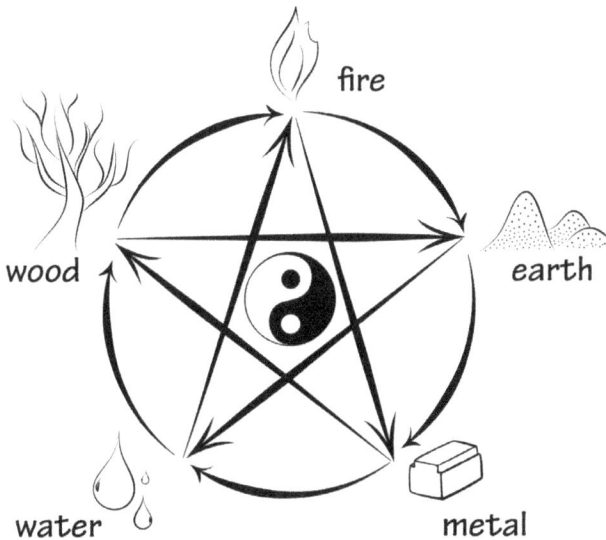

1. Water Element—Connection to Water

The presence of water will create a relaxed atmosphere that enhances qualities of communication and intuition. The water element is represented in materials such as water, glass, crystals, and free flowing patterns. Water element shapes are irregular, curving, flowing, and winding. Irregular shapes create a free and fluid motion that inspires the mind to wander.

In Feng Shui, water represents prosperity and the emotion of fear. Humans are made up primarily of the water elements, and so water is essential to life. Fix any water leaks, drips, and blocks immediately. Balancing water is critical to our innate primal self.

Activate the water element with clean, gentle flowing water to bring in peace and prosperity. Remove all stagnant and dirty water, and fountains that do not work.

> Colors: black, navy blue
> Shapes: irregular, curving, flowing, winding
> Materials: water, glass, crystal, free flowing forms and patterns

2. Wood Element—Connection to Wood/Tree

The wood element has an upward moving dynamic that encourages qualities of growth, flexibility, and creativity. The presence of wood creates an immediate connection to nature and encourages change and movement. The wood element is all around us and is seen as herbs, plants, flowers, fruit, trees, and any type of wood or paper product. Bring live healthy plants into your home and avoid all dried flowers, as they have no life force. Plants such as the peace lily can clean the air and help remove the negative effects of electromagnetic fields. Connect to powerful plant symbology to attract financial gain: the jade plant has leaves that resemble coins, and is called the money plant of Feng Shui. Bamboo also represents prosperity, as it grows with flexibility, and in sections for strength.

> Colors: green, purple, soft blue
> Shape: rectangle
> Materials: wood, paper, plants, trees, flowers

3. Fire Element—Connection to Fire

Here comes the sun! The fire element lights up our lives. The qualities of fire are inspiration, enlightenment, clarity, expression, passion and intelligence. The fire element is represented by the sun, all forms of fire, candles, lighting, animals, animal products, and human beings. The triangular flame shape of the fire element excites and elevates. It creates drama, high energy, and tension. Fire must be handled with care! The fire element should not be overused in areas such as bedrooms, counseling rooms, and quiet gathering rooms because it creates too much activity and yang

energy. In primal times, we used fire to cook our food, and it of-
fered protection from the dark night. We gathered around the fire
for warmth and ceremony. Fire brings us hope and inspiration to
create our visions.

Colors: red, orange
Shape: triangle, pyramid
Material: fire, candles, animals, humans

4. Earth Element—Connection to Earth

The Earth element is truly the foundation that we all stand upon.
Earth qualities express as stability, reliability, honesty, and support. The very stable shape of a square is the form of the earth element. Squares promote a feeling of grounding and safety. Square
buildings feel safe and sturdy. Humans have a primal need to feel
safe and stable, and so the earth element is critical and foundational. Too much earth can discourage creativity and individuality, so use the earth as a base to bring stability into your environment. Bring the earth element into children's bedrooms using
flooring options that create a sense of gravity and grounding. Use
natural earth materials for home décor such as slate, brick, and
clay. Square shaped dining tables are highly desirable in Feng
Shui as a way to create balance and grounding.

Colors: yellow, brown, beige
Shape: square
Materials: soil, clay, marble, brick, sand

5. Metal Element—Connection to Metal

Bringing it all together is the metal element. Metal qualities are
about being ethical, focused, organized, logical, gathering, and
completing. The shape of metal is round like a coin or a circle.
Round shapes encourage conversation and equality. A round table creates balanced conversations. When gathering around a fire
in a circle, the circle represents unity and solidarity. One of the
most famous circles is the Round Table where the knights came
to unite and pledge allegiance to a higher purpose.

The metal element allows us to feel connected to our tribe,

ourselves, and honors the circle of life. Use a round table in the kitchen to generate communication and informal camaraderie. All are equal around the round table.

Colors: white, gray, silver, gold, copper
Shape: circle
Materials: iron, steel, copper, silver, gold, all metals

Lesson Three

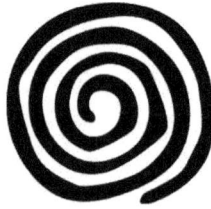

LESSON THREE: LOCATION, LOCATION, LOCATION
Land, Placement, Location, Surroundings

Today, we do not often think of a location as a life/death choice, yet in primal times, making a poor choice for your home base could be life threatening. Ideal locations are sheltered from extreme weather, floods, decaying land, and landslides.

Ideally, we choose a property that has life-enhancing qualities, such as nearby resources, friendly neighbors, quality water and air, food, connection. As we discovered in learning the qualities of the five elements, shapes have different qualities and dynamics. Lot shapes, roadways, and other topographical features will dictate the safety and success of our homes.

We must consider the components of the land shape that we are "claiming" as ours. The best shapes for a property lot is a square or a rectangle. Squares and rectangles are balanced and symmetrical. An irregular water shaped lot can have unstable boundary issues. The most difficult lot shape is the fire element shaped lot. The triangle, shaped like a flame, brings instability, sudden events, and drama.

What is the topography of the property? Ideally, we seek a home location that has a slightly elevated landform behind it to reinforce power and protect the "back" of our domain. In Feng Shui teachings the elevated hill behind a space is called the "Black Turtle." A home that has a drop behind it experiences a loss of power, prosperity, and relationships. A flat piece of property can create a "turtle hill" by reinforcing the back property with fencing—stone, wood, tall plantings.

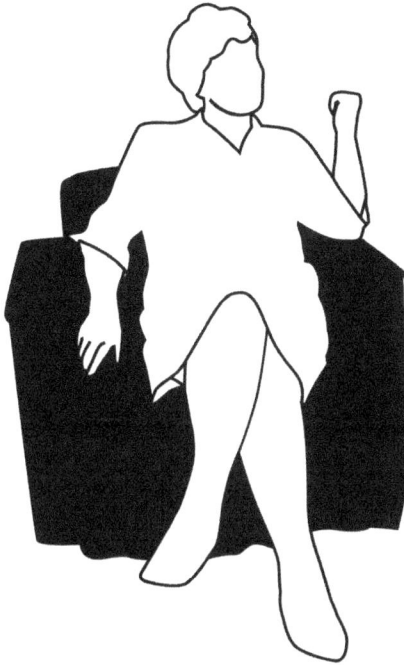

This ancient dynamic of the armchair shape is the foundation of Form School Feng Shui—the first formalized teaching.

The armchair formation is a primal configuration that we naturally embody at every opportunity. The basic rules are: Keep your back protected. Have a clear unobstructed view of what is in front of you.

A home that is located too close to the road experiences opportunity that flies by, and never comes to the door. Homes are best centrally located on the land, having some road frontage for protection and welcome and a large backyard for personal power and privacy. A home that is situated below the road level subjects the house to unsafe conditions such as negative water and ice flow. Living in a home below road level creates a daily flow against gravity. As we leave our home, we have to climb out and this creates stress and a feeling that it is a big effort to go into the world daily.

Location, Location, Location

A home with an excess of water behind it can diminish strength and power. Water represents prosperity, financial issues, emotional stress, and psychic influences. A beautiful water fountain will activate prosperity and is best placed in the front center of the house exterior or the back left of the property. Those two locations connect with the water element and allow water to create support and flow.

Water holds memory and is very interactive with the home dynamics. All water drips, blocks, and floods signify financial and emotional concerns. Fix all unbalanced water immediately. Ponds especially can create an issue when they become stagnant.

In Feng Shui, the back center of the property is the fire element and represents future money. When water is placed in this location, we experience a clash of elements, and water will "put out" the fire. This happens often when swimming pools are located in the back center of the property. This is a great area for a fire pit! The fire element in Feng Shui represents how the world sees you, treats you, and respects you. Are you being paid what you are worth?

Your placement of your home on your lot will also inflence the energy you attract. A home that is placed too close to the road has a challenging time attracting and holding opportunity. A car flies by rapidly and misses the home/business completely and the driver says, "Oops, missed that one!" A home at the very end of a long road, a dead end, or a tight cul-de-sac, can feel oppressed.

Tips:
* Look for plot shapes that are balanced, such as a square or rectangle.
* Seek property with a small hill or rise in the back.
* Avoid stagnant water on the property.
* Choose a home that is at ground level or higher, not a drop below the road.
* Place a home a safe distance from the road, creating a buffer between road and house.

Lesson Four

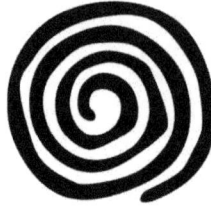

LESSON FOUR: FANGS, POINTS AND BLADES

As human beings, we respond negatively when a pointed object is directed at us. This is a primal survival response. Sometimes a knife or a pair of scissors might not be pointed directly at you, as points can be hidden or subtle such as when sitting in the direct path of the pointed edge of a wall.

Let us consider a ceiling fan that is directly above the bed. The conscious mind will look at it and think, "What if that ever fell?" and then respond internally with the statement, "That is silly, that would never happen." We dismiss the concern. As the conscious mind sleeps, the subconscious primal mind is on alert watching the dangerous blades above. Sleep becomes restless and disturbed, and there is an underlying sense of anxiety and danger.

A poison arrow is a Feng Shui term for sharp points that point toward us to create a stabbing effect. We could be sitting or lying next to a pointed wall corner edge, a file cabinet corner, a corner of a bedroom dresser, or end table, or window blinds with pointed blades that "chop into the room." We live with many points and edges that we ignore or dismiss. Yet the primal mind has been alerted and will watch these threats.

The body becomes alerted to danger, and the area of the body that is feeling "attacked" will activate, warn, and stress. Ongoing stress can lead to aches, pains, and discomfort. Curved furniture and rounded edges naturally bring our primal instincts to peace.

Tips:

* First, do a "blade" check of the home. Look at areas where you spend a lot of time sitting, sleeping, eating.
* Ceiling fans—we love our ceiling fans, as they move the energy around and circulate flow. To reduce the "threatening" fan blades, paint the ceiling white. Get a low-profile style white ceiling fan that will "disappear" into the design. A Feng Shui "cure" is to attach a round clear crystal to the fan as well.
* For end tables near the bed, add a decorative cloth to the top of the table, softening the edges. If you have edges and points from walls and file cabinets coming towards you, move them or move your location so as not to be affected by the points.
* Blinds can have very sharp edges. It is recommended to keep blinds open or closed. Better yet, change out the blinds to a softer style. Highly recommended is a bottom-up style shade that can be adjusted to the lower window, upper window, or cover it all. This makes for an optimal experience of safety.

Lesson Five

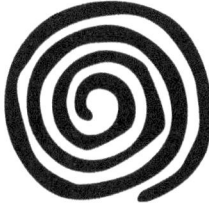

LESSON FIVE: DANGER FROM ABOVE

As we tune into our primal instincts, we begin to experience our homes in a new way. Our next lesson will look at the influence of "danger from above," or the experience of beams, low ceilings and pressure from above.

Ancient Asian systems represent man's journey on Earth as a threefold experience. With proper balance and connection, man's ideal experience on Earth is called "Heaven on Earth for Man." Man stands on the Earth, and above him is Heaven. Earth is our foundation, our home. Heaven is seen as the "sky," our future, the ability to reach unhindered and unlimited toward our highest potential. In our homes, our ceilings represent our sky or heaven and are also symbolic of our "future." Honoring the law of gravity, we stand on the stable ground and are able to feel the openness and expansion of the space above us. Ceiling height has an impact on the energy we experience in our home. A ceiling that is too low is both oppressive and smothering. A ceiling that is a dark color creates the feeling of a dark future ahead. A ceiling that is too high can cause a feeling of vulnerability, over-exposure and a loss of grounding and security. Rooms that have vaulted ceilings are beautiful, yet are often avoided as they lack intimacy.

Ceiling beams are a design trend that make a bold statement, bringing a sense of drama into a home. Ceiling beams also create a heavy weight over our heads, especially when over a bed, table or a couch that is used often. Beams can chop and divide. Beams over a bed can divide a couple or apply weight across a part of the body. The lower the beams, the more the primal mind sees this as an oppressive threat.

Tips:

* To remedy a room with vaulted ceilings add some grounded earth toned furniture.
* Add a horizontal design line around the room—a border or a series of artwork.
* Add curtains that lower the line of the room.
  To remedy low ceilings use light colored walls.
* Use uplighting and lighting to lighten up the room.
* To remedy heavy, imposing ceiling beams paint the dark beams white, the same color as the ceiling.
* Avoid having any beams over a bed or dining table.

Lesson Six

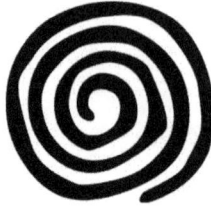

LESSON SIX: INVADING ENEMIES AND ENERGIES
Openings and Doorways

Doorways are openings and passageways that allow entry of chi into our homes. The exterior can be seen as the outside world. Once we go through the doorway, we transition into the personal interior space of the home. Doorways are important, and in Feng Shui they represent the parents—the authority of the family. Doors maintain our protection and our privacy.

Connecting back to our primal past, we know that doors are openings that can bring in the entrance of invading enemies, animals, and cold weather. Thus, entrances are not the safest position for our valuables. Where would you place your family, food, and resources in your home for the most protection? The ideal position for the most protection of valuables would be toward the back of the house. Most traditional tribal homes placed the children to the very back of the space for protection. Often dogs were placed near the entrance for added protection.

When entering a bedroom, we would seek the command position for the bed. The command position is the "farthest from the door, with a full view of the door." Where would you place a young vulnerable baby in their nursery?

As the place of intimacy, rest, romance, relaxation, and total vulnerability, the bedroom has a huge effect on our lives. When we close our eyes, we need to feel safe.

If we are sleeping in a compromised position, our primal instincts remain on alert and we remain in a "flight or fight" status. Bring support into the bedroom with a solid headboard. A solid headboard offers strong support and protects the head.

Avoid having a mirror reflect yourself in the bed. Seeing your reflection in bed creates an unsettling and startling dynamic. In Feng Shui it also attracts and doubles the number of people in the relationship.

Tips:

* Maintain a strong and powerful front door to set the tone of the home.
* Always keep doors unblocked.
* Align beds to the command position for the most support and protection.
* Have a strong solid wood headboard for the ideal protection and support.
* Avoid a mirror reflecting you in bed.

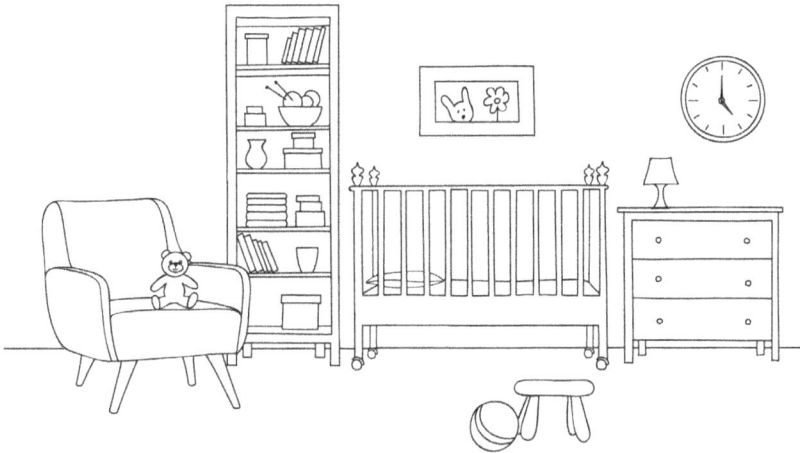

Lesson Seven

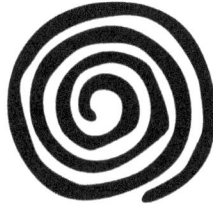

LESSON SEVEN: EVIL LURKS IN THE CORNERS
Dark and Hidden Areas

We are naturally programmed to avoid dark, secretive, and hidden areas. The unknown and nighttime were dangerous—many predators hunted at night with keen vision and scent. It was not safe to enter the darkness without fire to light the way and adequate protection.

Our homes are a representation of our lives. When we have rooms that are empty, unused, avoided, and cluttered, it shows us areas in our lives that we have not addressed or healed. The basement represents the past, the main floor represents the present time, and the attic and second floor represent the future. What levels of the house are cluttered, dark, and unused?

What is the story of your home? Where do you see stagnant and blocked areas? When areas are stagnant and dark in a home, they attract stale, unwanted, heavy energy. You may notice that children will avoid areas that are dark and ominous as a natural protective instinct. An excess of antiques and heavy, upholstered furnishings will contribute to the heavy atmosphere. Homes that have a history of divorce, arguments, illness, trauma and death hold onto the negative predecessor template creating areas that feel sad, angry and dark.

We avoid walking down dark streets and pathways. We avoid entering dark rooms. The placement of street lighting has a measurable effect in reducing crime. A college campus usually has adequate lighting throughout the school's paths and dorm areas. At home lighting makes our interior rooms feel inviting and larger. When we create adequate lighting options for all areas of

Evil Lurks in the Corners

our homes on all levels, we symbolize lighting up all areas of our life. We can move easily throughout each corner of our homes and properties with comfort and ease.

Creating illumination and access throughout our space is vital for a sense of safety and security, resolving a primary response trigger.

Tips:

Walk through all of your land, boundary to boundary to access your comfort level.

Utilize all your rooms, give them purpose.

Remove clutter

Place proper lighting in all rooms on all levels.

Walk through your home and notice how you feel in each area and level of your home. and adjust accordingly.

Lesson Eight

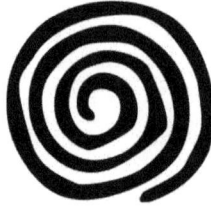

LESSON EIGHT: MEANDERING CHI— ROOM FLOW

Chi is defined as *Prana, Ki,* and *Life Force.* It is the essence of all living beings. Law #2 states that "Everything is alive with Energy," which means that everything is alive with chi.

We want our homes to invite in all the positive benefits of this life force and to create a beautiful meandering flow of energy throughout the entire home and into every room. From the moment you step over the threshold of your home, you will begin to move into and through your space. How does your home flow? If you have a bi-level home, you will immediately have to make a choice to go "up" or "down" steps. This split entry is called a Mandarin Duck entry, or a divorce style home entry because the message is always "split, divide, choose." Is the home plan welcoming and open, or is it choppy, closed and congested? When we enter a home easily and effortlessly, our mind and body are at ease. There are no stairs to climb or decisions to make. This creates a natural flow of chi that is easy to follow and which feels best to the primal brain.

The optimal dynamic is to locate public areas toward the front of the home and private areas toward the back of the space. Both in traditional Feng Shui and primal Feng Shui, the back of your home represents your power place and the area that can best hold and protect your most valuable resources. The best place for the master bedroom, kitchen, and dining room are locations in the back of the home where they can anchor power, protection and support.

Hallways and corridors are long passages through the home. Narrow, dark hallways drop our energy and create an un-

40

safe feeling within us. Lots of angles and sharp turns can create the feeling of danger "around the corner." Use light paint colors and adequate lighting in hallways, stairwells, and corridors. You can also use uplifting and positive artwork along the hallways to slow the fastmoving energy and create a positive flow.

Separating parents and children's bedrooms was a big design trend for years but ideally, family sleeping areas are best when located close to each other. It is a natural arrangement for protection and inner peace. Our primal instincts are to preserve ourselves and our families, and disjointed sleeping areas cause sleeplessness and stress.

Tips:

* With split staircases, always guide the eye up, never down.
* Add color and artwork to the top level bringing the chi and lifeforce up and into the main floor of the home.
* Unify the paint color through the home to make areas feel connected.
* Light up dark hallways.
* Use uplifting and natural artwork around the home.
* Add a touch lamp to a child's room for easy lighting access to increase their feeling of security.
* Place the photos of parents into the children's bedrooms for a feeling of safety and connection.

Lesson Nine

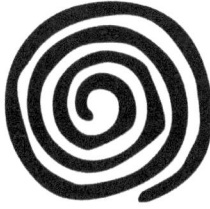

LESSON NINE: COLOR MY WORLD

Imagine a world without color. Color has a deep effect on humans, plants, and animals. It is the light language of the Earth, and it is deeply essential to life. Color can be influenced by country, culture, family, sports, experiences, and internal dynamics. We all have personal color preferences from our own experiences and energetic expression.

I certainly want to encourage you to express yourself colorfully. I am also going to share some insight concerning the power of color and the way it can influence you, especially in your home and office spaces. When we use color with purpose and intention, we become masters of our own environment. Understanding the primal color concepts that reside deep within us allows us to build a powerful foundational support system in our homes.

Let us explore the universal energies of colors and tap into the primal and foundational color messages that can bring our spaces to a place of safety and security. Primal color influence resides deep within our human DNA; cultural color influence is environmental, and personal color influence can be internal and reflect our conscious life interactions.

Surrounding ourselves with the harmonics of color
Colors and their meanings

Red: Fire element, primal, love, passion, lust, the color of blood. Anger, aggression, danger, action, energy, power, strength, heat Red always gets our attention.

Let us take a look at the color red. Red is a color that brings about action, passion, hunger, stimulation, blood pressure elevation, heat, and also anger. It is a color that is exalted in Asian cultures as a symbol of good luck—red envelopes are given for prosperity, health, and good luck at the beginning of each new year. In primal times, red was seen when blood was spilled. The blood of a menstrual cycle, was a sign of life. The blood of a hunted animal kill, was a sign of death. Blood is the liquid life force and essence that courses through the veins of living creatures.

Red is the color of fire: essential in life, it represents heat, warmth, protection, and also danger. Uncontrolled fire can take life, as easily as it can support life. Red is also the color of a cardinal and a ruby gemstone.

Red always commands attention. The color red is powerful and its effects can be both positive and negative. Red is essential to our lives—it offers action, inspiration, passion, and warmth. Use the color red with purpose in your homes and do not overuse it. In my many years of consultations and design work, I have witnessed red used excessively in homes, including red carpets in children's bedrooms, red bedrooms, and red kitchens. Living with an overflow of red creates overstimulation and activation, hyperactivity, and a good dose of anger. Avoid red in children's bedrooms. Add red when you need activity and stimulation. How much red is too much red? When your level of activity, heat and stimulation reaches a boiling point, then it is time to tone down the red.

Red Tips:
*   Bring touches of red into the master bedroom for passion and warmth. This could be two red roses, red hearts, or red accent pillows.
*   Add red to activity rooms, family rooms and children's play rooms.
*   Bring red to the office to activate sales, fame, and action. Enhance appetite and action by accenting red in the kitchen. with table and decor accents, red fruits, flowers.

Brown: Earth element, grounded, stable, safety, natural, honest, warm, dependable, reliable, comforting, balanced square shape. Brown is a color that connects us directly to the earth. The many colors of earth are: brown, sand, beige, clay—all introduce a feeling of support and stability. One of my favorite formulas for children's rooms is called "Gravity Design" that follows the flow of nature in the room. This is achieved with earth toned flooring (earth below), white ceilings (heaven above), and walls that are a soft green to encourage growth and healing.

Avoid too much brown as it can cause a person to be stuck, become narrow minded and get stagnant or blocked. Brown can make you play it "safe" and limit risk and independence.

Brown Tips:
* Use brown to create a stable grounded flooring into children's rooms.
* Brown is considered a dementia-friendly color and a good choice for room décor.
* Use brown decor in areas that feel too overactive and scattered.
* Brown, beige and earth toned walls are grounding and supportive.
* Utilize brown in bedrooms, living rooms, meditation rooms, dining rooms

Yellow: Earth element, our external and internal sun. Joy, happiness, hope, positivity, intelligence, clarity, health, youthful fear, cowardice, a noticeable, warning color Yellow is a color that evokes a reaction—we either like yellow or dislike it. Nature offers us many beautiful yellow flowers ,such as sunflowers and daffodils. It represents sunshine and the summer. Yellow can also be a warning color, as seen in a yellow traffic light and yellow warning signs. In nature the yellow and black stripes on bees get our attention and offer a clear warning sign. Yellow is a powerful memory enhancer. It has been used in products such as yellow highlighters and yellow note pads for intentional brain connection. Yellow has many diverse cultural interpretations.

In China, yellow was considered an imperial color of royalty and importance. In the Feng Shui home symbology, yellow is the symbol of health and the center of all life. The color yellow can stimulate the brain and bring up negative emotions, and is best avoided in bedrooms and in spaces for older adults.

Yellow Tips:
* Use yellow in a kitchen, dining room and living room.
* Use yellow to increase appetite.
* Use yellow to enhance memory.
* Use yellow for healing and health.
* Use yellow for mental clarity, wealth and attention.

Green: Wood element, healing, growth, upward moving, expansive, harmony, safety, wealth, youth, fertility, relaxing, greed, jealousy, lack of experience, illness.

Primal man was immersed with the color green, a color that dominates and connects us to nature and life force. We think of green trees and plants, fields and forests. Green represents the heart chakra and the healthy heart; it also represents the growth from seed to plant, an expression of the everlasting cycle of recreation and survival.

Green can also be calming, cooling, and healing. There are many shades of green: some are light and calming, some are bright and activating, and some are deep and grounded. Green is used as a color of positivity and forward movement. Green traffic lights tell us to "go."

Green plants represent the dynamic of wealth and prosperity. Avoid green when people are struggling with cancer and tumor growth, as green stimulates growth. Green is a positive color for children's bedrooms as it encourages and stimulates growth. Master bedrooms are best supported with earth tones for connection and grounding; the color green is not recommended for a master bedroom.

Green Tips:
* * Use green in children's bedrooms to encourage growth.
* * Use green in the kitchen and dining room.
* * Use green in meditation rooms, choosing a soft sage green.
* * Use green in living rooms.
* * Use green to activate creativity and stimulation.

Blue: Blue can be expressed as both the water and wood elements depending on the tones. Very deep blue—navy blue is aligned with the water element. Soft light blue is represented by the wood element. Blue creates individuality, serenity, wisdom, stability; calming, cooling, trust, loyalty, security, expansiveness; it encourages depression, and sadness. Too much blue can make us "blue."

When we seek blue in nature, all we need to do is look up. Blue is the color of the sky, our heaven above, our future. Blue is also seen in the many shades of water around the world—turquoise seas, green/blue ponds, blue water. Culturally, blue is seen as a spiritual color, the color of the Virgin Mary and Krishna. Avoid the color blue in the master bedroom, as it is "cooling" to the relationship. Avoid blue in dining rooms and restaurants as it inhibits appetite. Avoid dark blue in bathrooms and bedrooms as it creates excessive water energy.

Blue Tips:
* * Use a blue to create a calm atmosphere.
* * Use blue in meditation areas.
* * Paint light blue on walls in children's rooms.
* * Use blue in areas that need to feel "cool" and "calm."

Pink: Earth element, love, heart, mother, sweetness, feminine, playfulness, youthful, fun, compassion. Life is sweeter when we connect with the color pink. We can find pink in a gentle sunset or pink clouds in the twilight sky.

Pink speaks to the heart and creates a feeling of happiness and comfort that is as grounded as a mother's hug. The color pink relieves anger and aggression. Feeling "in the pink" is a sign of happiness and health. Bubble gum pink relieves stomach distress and has been used in popular antacid coloring.

Pink Tips:

* Use pink in children's rooms.
* Use pink in rooms for the elderly.
* Use pink when harmony is a goal.
* Use pink with the intention to dissipate anger.

Orange: Bright orange connects to the fire element, and darker terra cotta tones connect to the earth element. Orange creates unity, connection, fusion, creativity, friendship, happiness, release of grief, extroverted energy, fun, enthusiasm. It represents youth, a feeling of safety, and a zest for life.

Orange is a color that creates attention, commands attraction and always evokes a response. Orange is a powerful color tool in releasing the trauma of grief. Orange fruits are both uplifting and healing. We notice orange.

Orange encourages unity and thinking with "one mind"—a popular color of the Tibetan monks. Orange discourages independent thinking, so it is best to avoid orange when individuality is your goal. Orange is best avoided in offices where creative thinking is needed.

Orange Tips:

* Use orange in kitchens and dining rooms.
* Use orange in playrooms and living areas.
* Use peach toned oranges in bedrooms for single adults.
* Use orange for happiness and joy during the frosty winter months.
* Use orange when joy and happiness is needed.

Purple: Purple is associated with the wood element that re resents abundance. The color purple is spiritual, royal, representing wealth and luxury. It causes elevation and has a mysrerious aspect to it.

Purple has many beautiful shades from the dark regal purple of royalty to the soft lavender of meditation areas. In nature, we find the color purple in rich berries and fruit, and beautiful fields of lavender. Purple causes elevation as it connects us to our higher intelligence and spirituality. Avoid purple in kitchens and dining rooms as it limits appetite. Avoid purple in master bedrooms because it diminishes one's sexual appetite!

Purple Tips:
* Use purple in meditation rooms and healing spaces.
* Use soft purple in children's rooms.
* Use purple to activate wealth and abundance.

Gray: The color gray is represented as the metal element. Gray represents the father, control; it is practical, professional, conventional. It causes balance, receptivity, reserve, stability, safety. It helps one become smart, financially wise, serious,

The color gray is midpoint between black and white, and represents a balance of those extreme dynamics. Gray can be seen in natural stone and boulders. Gray is a very mature, dependable color and it became a decorating theme of the 2000s. Although gray is a safe and stable color, it can create a cold, unemotional template for a home when overused. Avoid it in bedrooms. Avoid where illness or depression is a concern.

Gray Tips:
* Use gray conservatively to create stability, safety, support.
* Use gray in offices to convey professionalism and stability.
* Use gray colors or natural stones to create a feeling of stability.

White: White is the metal element. The color white represents purity, cleanliness, perfection, innocence, faith, simplicity, minimalism, and sophistication. White fluffy clouds portray an image of cleanliness, innocence, and purity. Although white light contains all colors, we "see" white as a lack of color.

White can offer us an opportunity to have fresh, open space, a blank canvas—to invite in new ideas and stimulation. White has many cultural expressions. In the west, white is the color of the bride's wedding gown—her symbol of purity and innocence and new beginnings. In many countries, white represents the color of death and mourning.

Avoid overusing white, as it will create a cold and emotionless atmosphere. Avoid white in the master bedroom as a main color, and in bedding. The master bedroom is our most intimate space, and the ideal colors are those connected to the human skin tones—rose, cream, cocoa, brown, beige, pink. In the master bedroom, white is seen as sterile and cold.

White Tips:
* Use white to create an open, cool, fresh atmosphere.
* Use white as an accent color to highlight colors.
* Use white as a backdrop for areas with a large amount of artwork.
* Use white in kitchens to create a clean, fresh feeling.

Black: Black is the water element. The color black represents elegance, depth, sophistication, protection, power, luxury, darkness, depression, mystery, danger, abyss, and evil.

The blackness of night, or a dark deep cave bring an air of mystery and danger. What cannot be seen is an unsafe situation for humans.

The color black represents the deep dark water element of our birth—from dark into light. Black can offer a form of protection and is a favorite color of urban New Yorkers. Black is worn as a color of mourning and respect in many cultures. It is also a color of formal attire and elegance. When we see a red cardinal, a blue bluebird, a yellow finch, we feel inspired and uplifted. When we see a black crow or raven, we feel a sense of mystique, awe and intimidation. The black colored bird commands our attention.

Black is a powerful color to be used for drama, depth, and attention in a deeper, darker, mystical way. Black can also create coldness and depression when overused. It does not allow focus or enlightenment but can call us down into the abyss. The dark tones bring an excess of water when overused in rooms. Avoid black in the kitchen and dining room as it creates an overly formal atmosphere. White is the best kitchen color allowing the colors of the food to shine. Avoid black in hallways and stairways; a black passageway does not invite uplift or safety.

Black Tips:

* Use black as an accent color for drama and attention.
* Use black to create a sophisticated theme.
* Use black as an accent wall for drama and depth.

Embrace the gift of color and consciously bring color symbolism into your space to affect your psychology. Honor the primal ancestry and DNA of your color coding and avoid what is the latest trend and design statement. Always create grounding, connection, and balance.

Lesson Ten

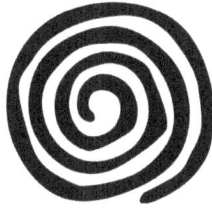

LESSON TEN: GATHER WITH ME
Kitchens and Dining Rooms

The kitchen is often designed as the official "heart of the home." It is the area where people tend to stand, gather, chat, and watch the cook prepare the meal. It is the area where we sit with a friend over a cup of tea or coffee. We can trace the intoxicating scent of chocolate chip cookies into the kitchen and watch them coming out of the oven toasted brown and bubbly. The kitchen holds our food, our source of nourishment and life.

According to ancient Feng Shui wisdom, the stove is the prime representative of health and wealth, and is honored as such. When we have the ability to feed ourselves, we are truly wealthy. The stove represents survival and success. Stove condition, location and cleanliness are key components in a healthy home. The primal fire, the source of ancient nourishment, is represented by today's stove.

Dining rooms are where we gather around a table with our family to share a meal which is the ultimate expression of love and abundance. In primal times, the gathering and dining would have been around a fire, where food was prepared and then shared. Today, a round or circle shaped table creates a natural dynamic that invites equality and stimulates conversation. A rectangular table represents the wood element. For dining, it is a formal shape, with a "king" and "queen" chair at both ends of the table. The rectangular table is wonderful for traditional family gatherings, holidays, and important occasions.

"Gather With Me"

Tips:

* Avoid all clutter in the kitchen and dining room.
* Ideally, white is the best color in a kitchen to highlight cleanliness and display food.
* Keep the stove in prime condition, making sure all burners are working.
* Keep the stove immaculate and shining, as it represents wealth and health.
* Avoid eating in the living room or family room.
* Set a table of invitation both in the kitchen and dining areas.

Lesson Eleven

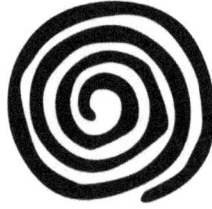

LESSON ELEVEN: UNITY AND CONNECTION
Living and Family Rooms

Creating rooms that invite our family and friends to share and connect is a key component in creating balanced spaces. Family rooms are usually casual whereas living rooms have a formal atmosphere in which outside guests and family are invited to spend an evening. The living room defines the theme and personality of the home. Artwork, color, textures, and light create invitation. Avoid having individual televisions or computers in bedrooms as this encourages separation.

Create activities for each family member to enjoy in your family room. It is still as vital today, as it was in primitive times, to stay connected with each other and to create space for a gathering and for unity. Human connection is a vital part of humanity and a base, primal need.

Tips:

* Remove excess clutter from your living areas.
* Create a fun family room atmosphere where each person in the family is acknowledged.
* Keep the seating areas open and welcoming and not blocked.
* Avoid sharp edges on coffee tables and furniture.
* Use inviting colors and fabrics for inspiration and connection.

Lesson Twelve

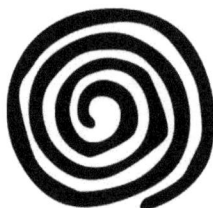

LESSON TWELVE: OUR NEST—BEDROOMS

In Feng Shui, bedrooms have the greatesst influence on our life force. The bedroom is a place where we are the most vulnerable—here we close our eyes and go into deep sleep. If the body feels completely safe and secure, then the rest is peaceful and beneficial. If the room has negative features, then the primal mind keeps a part of us on "alert," ready for fight or flight.

All bed positions are best when out of the direct path of the door. Finding a strong command position is vital—the farthest from the door, while maintaining view of the door. Many young children do well when one side of the bed is along a wall for extra support and protection. The bed can be adjusted as they mature and grow. All bedrooms require a solid headboard, preferably made of wood or material in a solid calming color. Headboards protect the vulnerable head area and symbolize having support in life. The headboard needs to be attached to the bed, and not the wall.

Children's bedrooms do well with a calming color scheme, utilizing soft greens for growth, and earth toned flooring for stability. Pictures of parents and loved ones bring a sense of protection to children. Having a lamp accessible within reach is important. Avoid overstimulation with loud sheets, blankets and toy clutter. Avoid bunk beds as they create pressure for the child.

The purpose of the master bedroom is to support us with rest, relaxation, romance and rejuvenation. Consider your bedroom to be your sanctuary, where you can finally let your guard down—here we can close our eyes and let go.

Things to avoid in your master bedroom—too many mirrors, a work desk, exercise equipment, pictures of family, and most of all—clutter ! When we see a work desk in our bedroom, our thoughts immediately think about work. Exercise equipment, ironing boards, clutter – all of these items create distraction from the bedroom's main purpose of rest, romance and rejuvenation. Remember Law #2, *Everything is Alive with Energy*? When we have pictures of family members, parents, and children in our bedrooms, we are inviting their living energy into our most intimate space. The bedroom is only for you and your partner. It is your room for recovery and intimacy.

The ideal colors for the master bedroom are all the beautiful skin tones—connecting us to our body and creating a sense of grounding and security. These colors are: rose, pink, mauve, cream, beige, cocoa, and brown. Bring in artwork and photos that represent love and relationship.

Tips:

* Align the bed to its strongest room position—out of the direct pathway from the door.
* Choose a strong solid headboard; avoid a metal headboard. Choose wood or fabric.
* A queen size bed is the most auspicious for a master bedroom.
* Check for sharp points and edges.
* Remove fans or replace fans with a white low profile design.
* Clean up all clutter—use organizational systems that can be covered.
* Keep the television out of the bedrooms, as well as computers and phones.
* Have no more than one mirror in the bedroom and not in view of the bed.
* Remove all furniture that has a negative past and memory.

Lesson Thirteen

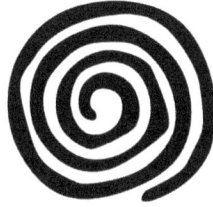

LESSON THIRTEEN: YOUR LIVING HOME
Spirit, Symbols, Signs

Are you connected to your home? Do you love it? Do you honor it?

Connecting to the Spirit of the Home

Our homes have a unique presence called the Spirit of the Home. It is the living essence and energy of the home. The Spirit of the Home is created when the home is built, and the roof and the front door are locked into place. This connection creates a birthday for the home. Many ancient cultures acknowledge the living presence of their home and honor their home with a beautiful altar and ceremony.

Home Theme

What is the essence of your home? When people enter your space, do they feel peaceful, stressed, or angry? Your home has an unspoken focus and theme. What does your home say?

Do you have pictures of children on every wall ? If so, the children basically run the energy of the house.

Are you the keeper of the family history and antiques? Then your ability to be seen and heard in the present time is overwhelmed by predecessor energy. If you are a collector, what do you collect? Your collections create an identity and tell a story.

Artwork, Statues, and Symbols

Artwork is a modern and powerful way to create an empowered

Your Living Home

template for your home. Each piece of art is a "living window," a view into reality, alive with living energy. Images of mountains bring in the energy of support and strength. Sunflowers bring in sacred geometry and create a feeling of harmony and balance. Avoid negative images of storms, chaos, and negative quotations.

Tips:
* Enter your home through the front door as often as possible to honor yourself and the home.
* Walk completely around your home, room to room, each level and notice if you find a theme.
* Set up an altar in the house as a place of respect, pause, and reflection.
* Organize photos and collections in specific areas, and not all over the house.
* Choose artwork, statues, symbols and photos of all that you love. Do not settle.
* Remove all items with negative memories and attachments.
* Remove all broken items, especially stopped clocks.
* Consider you home to be your vision board.

Lesson Fourteen

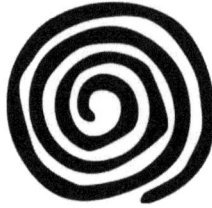

LESSON FOURTEEN: IT DOESN'T FEEL GOOD IN HERE
Space Clearing and Energy Maintenance

Land, color and décor only make up a part of our home template. The energy of the home, what is not visibly seen with the eye, plays a big part in how we feel in our space. Events, especially traumatic events will leave a tangible residue in the space. Anger, arguments, sadness, mental instability, and fear can stay in spaces through millennia unless specifically cleaned with space clearing.

Whether a home is a beautiful elaborate mansion or an old, dilapidated structure, there is an energetic template that resides in the home. This energy is made up of the Earth's ley lines, past residents, trauma and unresolved issues that have created a matrix in the space.

Honor your instincts. Feel your gut and tune into the actual "feeling" of your space. Does it feel heavy, sad, or angry? Energy maintenance and space clearing are necessary components to create a safe sanctuary and balanced space. Ancient primal homes used active fire as a part of their daily life for warmth, food preparation and protection. Fire and smoke are key elements in space clearing energetics. Through the centuries the burning of herbs such as sage and sweetgrass were implemented for space clearing. The space clearing process cleanses the home of the old matrix, and is thus reset with new intention. You do not have to use smoke or herbs to make a positive shift in your home. One of the most powerful processes you can do is to clear your home of all clutter.

Clearing clutter releases old stagnant chi, and creates an instant shift. Clutter is a complete block and is representative of "unfulfilled dreams."

Some of the effects of clutter are:
Disorganization
Creation of chaos
Activation of depression
Excess weight
Health problems
Staying stuck in the past
Sleeping disorders.

Energy maintenance and home cleansing will benefit you in many ways. Clearing out old patterns and predecessor energy from your space opens new possibilities. Predecessor energy is ancestral energy that is connected to the house and land from the past—former owners, tenants, builders, native people. Any trauma from predecessors will remain as an invisible dynamic unless resolved and cleared. Replacing a dark, heavy energy template with a new and bright one will increase your life force and vitality. You can activate your goals, uplift your spirits, and reclaim your space in a new and powerful way. Primal cultures practiced their own individual forms of space clearing, but all of them addressed the unseen energy of the land and home. Fire, smoke, salt, sound, herbs, oils, feathers, prayer, and ritual were the basis of all space clearing ceremonies.

Tips for some Simple Space Clearing Strategies:

* Remove clutter.
* Clean the space.
* Turn off electronics—televisions, computers
* Open doors and windows for one to two hours
* Use aromatherapy and essential oils to clear and uplift the space.
* Bring in fresh flowers, especially roses.
* Light candles.
* Walk through the space with smudging herbs such as sweetgrass and sage.
* Call in your spiritual assistants and prayers to set healing intentions.

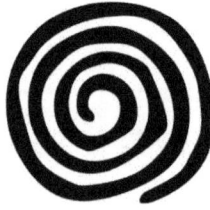

HOME AS A CIRCLE OF LIFE

Let us take a deeper look at the template of our homes starting with the traditional Feng Shui map called the *bagua*, and then at the primal Feng Shui model of the circle of life.

Traditional Feng Shui uses an analysis map called the *bagua*. It is an eight sided octagon that maps out the nine *guas* or houses of a home or space. The areas are Journey—Career and Inner Wisdom and Knowledge, Family and Ancestors, Prosperity and Abundance, Fame and Reputation, Relationship and Marriage, Children and Creativity, Helpful People and Travel, and to the Center—the Tai Chi. The *bagua* is a valuable tool in evaluating and adjusting any home or space to its highest potential. The *bagua* is applied to home and property plans.

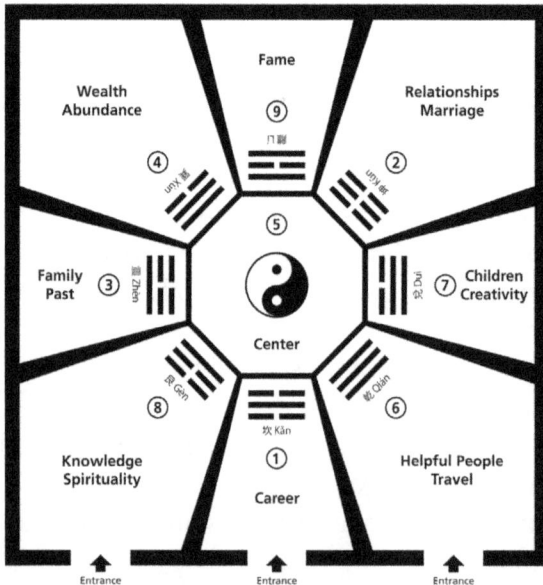

The *bagua* is aligned to the front door representing a first step into life's journey. Each gua represents an area of our life.

The *Guas* or Houses of the *Bagua* are:

Gua 1 : Career and Life Journey
Gua 2. Relationships/Marriage
Gua 3. Family, Ancestors
Gua 4. Wealth/Abundance
Gua 5. Center—combination of all
Gua 6. Helpful People, Travel
Gua 7. Children/Creativity
Gua 8. Knowledge, Inner wisdom
Gua 9. Fame, Fortune

Bagua Analysis: *Gua* by *Gua*
Gua 1: Career/Life Journey
Element: Water
Shape: Wavy
Trigram: Kan
Direction: North
Body Part: Ears
Family Member: Middle Son
Color: Black

The Career/Life Journey *Gua* represents your career, and what you bring to the world, including your skills and talents. As a water element, this area of the home needs to flow unhindered and unobstructed. Meandering movement is the desirable energy for this area. This house is a foundational house that brings your innate birthrights and wisdom into the world. The Career/Life Journey *Gua* is your life purpose. This area harmonizes with soft wavy shapes, the color black and water. Images of a soft gentle river will create a meandering flow of chi into the home. Clear crystals such as chandeliers represent the water element and make a beautiful enhancement for the home.

Gua 2: Relationships/ Marriage
Element: Earth
Shape: Square
Trigram: Kun
Direction: South-West
Body Part: Organs
Family Member: Mother
Color: Pink

The Marriage/Relationship *Gua* represents the dynamics and energy of relationships, the intimacy of two. In an office or commercial space, the relationship house represents intimate connection to one's staff, partners, and clients. This area holds the dynamic of mother, love, and commitment. This is the most feminine of the home sectors and carries an essence of warmth and caring. This area is best represented with symbols of two. Bring in pairs of two, such as two candles, two chairs, two lovebirds, etc.

Gua 3: Family/Ancestors, the past
Element: Wood – Thunder
Shape: Rectangle
Trigram: Chen
Direction: East
Body Part: Feet
Family Member: Eldest son
Color: Green

The Family/Ancestors *Gua* represents all issues related to our past ancestors, lineage, tribes, support groups, inner circles. At work, this area relates to your work family. This area holds the dynamics of your past connections. Family traditions, stories and trauma are represented here. This area relates to all people that have returned home to live. This area also connects to our animal family and is a place to honor our pets. The very active wood element is well represented in our homes with the color green and live plants and flowers.

Gua 4: Wealth/ Abundance
Element: Wood, Wind
Shape: Rectangle
Trigram: Sun
Direction: Southeast
Body Part: Pelvic area, Bones
Family Member: Eldest daughter
Color: Purple

The Wealth/Abundance *Gua* is often called the prosperity house or money corner. This is an area that invites in the chi (life force) of abundant flow. This is a place of power and resources in the home, and a great place to store your valuables and utilize symbols of wealth and prosperity. This area called the wind is about influencing others, and being influenced. It represents a time to branch into the world, build independence, seek adventure. In this home, this area attracts good luck. Activate the wood element with fresh plants, amethyst stones, and a gentle waterfall.

5: Center
Element: Considered Earth, but is a combination of all elements
Trigram: No Trigram; Yin/Yang is the symbol of the center
Shape: Square
Direction: Center
Body Part: Can represent all areas not in the other sectors, and all health issues.
Color: Yellow

The Center area oversees the balance and harmony of the space. It represents health. This area is the connection and center of all the other life houses in the *bagua* life map. A center is ideally always kept clutter free and clean. The center of a home is the connection point for all the other rooms and spaces. If you have a center staircase cutting through the center of the house, consider bringing in the earth element with earth tones of beige, brown, cream, and yellow to ground the center.

Gua 6: Helpful People/ Travel
Element: Metal, Heaven
Shape: Circle
Trigram: Chien
Direction: Northwest
Body Part: Head
Family Member: Father
Color: Gray

The Helpful People/ Travel *Gua* brings two dynamics to us. Helpful people represent all the people, mentors, and spiritual guides that come and assist you. It also asks that you become helpful to others to create balance. The travel aspect of this house represents all aspects of traveling: work, vacation, exploration. The very strong force of heaven in this area creates a sense of respect and authority. In the home, this is a metal area. Metal picture frames with pictures of your mentors, and helpful people, will create stability and support.

Gua 7: Children/Creativity
Element: Metal, Lake
Shape: Circle
Trigram: Tui
Direction: West
Body Part: Mouth/ Teeth/ Lungs
Family Member: Youngest daughter
Color: White

The Children/Creativity *Gua* represents the life force that we create in the world. This can represent children and creative projects. It is the energy of manifestation for the future. Fertility issues can be addressed within this house, looking at blocks, stagnancy, and emptiness symbolized in the home. Uplift this area with round and circular décor, such as a round mirror and round metal table. This sector can activate fun and playfulness, and a return to our inner child.

Gua 8: Knowledge/Inner Wisdom
Element: Earth, Mountain
Shape: Square
Trigram: Ken
Direction: North-East
Body Part: Hands
Family Member: Youngest son
Color: Blue

The Knowledge/Inner Wisdom *Gua* represents our journey into understanding who we are. This house has the dynamic of inner contemplation, education, wisdom, and self-reflection. Our self-awareness and inner cultivation opens the door to healthier relationships and opportunities. This house allows us to nurture ourselves like a seed that is able to transform from the inner to making our presence into the world. This symbolism of the mountain brings a sense of quiet, stillness, and a deep hidden strength to us. This is an ideal area for a meditation room or study. Place an empty vessel in this area to be your symbol of receptivity, such as an empty bowl or a vase.

Gua 9: Fame, Fortune
Element: Fire
Shape: Triangle
Trigram: Li
Direction: South
Body Part: Eyes
Family Member: Middle daughter
Color: Red

The Fame *Gua* is about your illumination in life. It represents your reputation, and how the world sees you. Are you being respected, acknowledged, and paid what you are worth? This area connects to joy, success and being seen in the light. This relates to the body part of the eyes, and everything connected with vision —seeing and being seen. Ignite passion, enthusiasm, and action.

Home as a Circle of Life

Intuition and clarity allow the inner light to be recognized in the outer world with brilliance. In our homes, this area resonates with a fireplace, fire pit, candles, lighting and triangular shapes.

Use this area to sketch your house:

Notes and observations about your home

What is the first thing you see when opening the door?

What areas are cluttered?

What are the rooms most utilized?

What are the rooms not used or used infrequently?

What are your additional observations on your home?

Let's do a Life Analysis—Gua by Gua—Life Sectors

Name _____ Today's Date _____

RATE EACH AREA FROM 1-10 with 10 being the highest

_____RATE YOUR HEALTH TODAY? Center *Gua*
_____RATE YOUR FAMILY'S HEALTH? Center *Gua*
_____DO YOU LOVE YOUR CAREER? Career/ Life Journey
Gua
_____RATE YOUR FLOW and LIFE JOURNEY Career/ Life
Journey *Gua*
_____ DO YOU CONTINUE TO LEARN? Inner Wisdom *Gua*
_____ DO YOU CREATE TIME FOR INNER CONTEMPLA-
TION? Inner Wisdom *Gua*
_____RATE YOUR RELATIONSHIP TO YOUR ANCESTRAL
FAMILY Family *Gua*
_____RATE YOUR RELATIONSHIP TO WORK AND SOCIAL
FAMILY Family *Gua*
_____WHAT IS YOUR CURRENT FINANCIAL HEALTH
Wealth *Gua*
_____DO YOU HOLD AND ACCUMULATE RESOURCES
Wealth *Gua*
_____DO YOU GET PAID WHAT YOU ARE WORTH? Fame
Gua
_____RATE HOW OTHERS SEE YOU, TREAT YOU AND
RESPECT YOU Fame *Gua*
_____RATE YOUR MARRIAGE OR INTIMATE
RELATIONSHIP Marriage *Gua*
_____RATE YOUR CLOSE WORK RELATIONSHIPS Marriage
Gua
_____RELATIONSHIP TO CHILDREN OR YOUR LIFE
PROJECTS Children *Gua*
_____RATE YOUR LEVEL OF FUN AND EXPRESSION
Children *Gua*
_____YOUR RECEIVING FROM HELPFUL PEOPLE Helpful

People *Gua*
_____ YOUR CONNECTION TO SPIRITUALITY Helpful
People *Gua*

Highest Point Total Possibility is 180 points.
My total is _____

What *Guas* or Life Areas rated the highest?

What *Guas* or Life Areas rated the lowest?

Apply the Life Analysis to your home with the Bagua Map, and note what rooms and house sectors scored the highest. In the areas with low ratings, note what the house is showing you. You may see clutter, stopped clocks, dripping faucets, empty rooms, etc. You home will mirror your current life situation. This is your opportunity to see your home as a vision board that can shift the blocked and stuck areas of your life. We want our homes to represent both our current time and our future visions.

Home as a Circle of Life

Our homes are a mirror of our personal life and our family dynamics. Our homes also represent our human journey as seen as the circle of life. The front of a home has an entry that allows transition from the *outside world* to the *inside world*. The front of a home is considered the public part of a home. The back of our home is our power place, a place where we place all of our valuables to safety and protection. Ideally sleeping areas, especially master bedrooms, kitchens, and family rooms are aligned along the back part of the home.

The Connection of the Bagua with the Circle of Life

The ancient Feng Shui bagua is in full alignment with the circle of life dynamic. The bagua offers a life view through the 9 sectors called guas. Our homes are a mirror of our life, and we can go one step further is following the chi, life force, in and through the home in a circular flow. The circle of life carries us through life's journey from birth through transition in a clockwise pattern.

The House as the Circle of Life:

From the entry way the energy follows life's journey as it travels clockwise through the house until it completes the circle around and back to the beginning.

1: Front Door: Entry into personal space and journey.
2. Inner Wisdom—Learning about the Self
3. Family and Ancestors—Growth, Forceful, Bright
4. Food, Resources, Water Supply—Prosperity
5. Power and Future Wealth—Fireplace—Fame
6. Marriage, Master Bedroom, Protected Mother
7 Children and Creative Energies, Mirror, Circle
8. Helpful People—Travel Realm to Realm, Transformation
Center—Core and Centralized Power Place

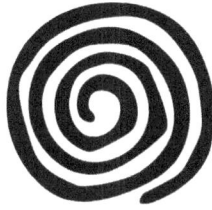

HOUSE AS A CIRCLE OF LIFE

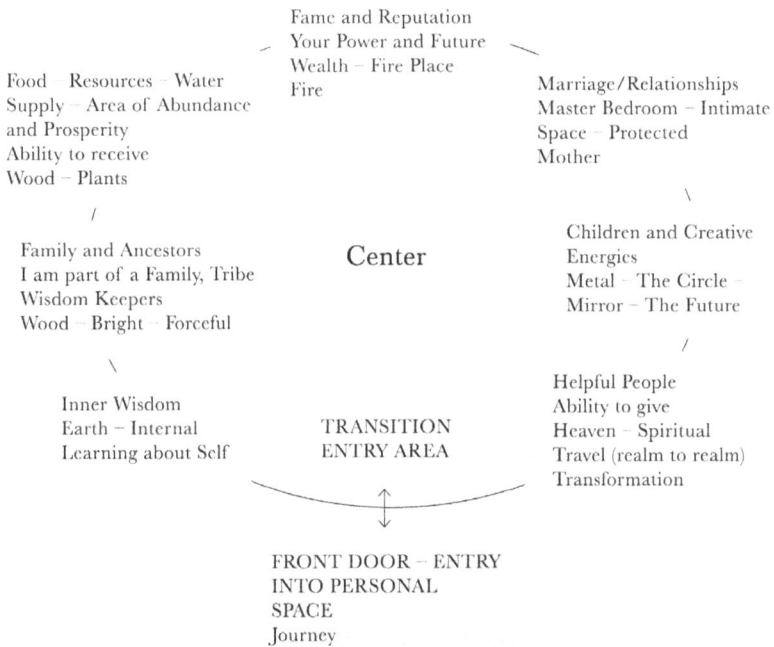

Fame and Reputation
Your Power and Future
Wealth – Fire Place
Fire

Food – Resources – Water
Supply – Area of Abundance
and Prosperity
Ability to receive
Wood – Plants

Marriage/Relationships
Master Bedroom – Intimate
Space – Protected
Mother

Family and Ancestors
I am part of a Family, Tribe
Wisdom Keepers
Wood – Bright – Forceful

Center

Children and Creative
Energies
Metal – The Circle –
Mirror – The Future

Inner Wisdom
Earth – Internal
Learning about Self

TRANSITION
ENTRY AREA

Helpful People
Ability to give
Heaven – Spiritual
Travel (realm to realm)
Transformation

FRONT DOOR – ENTRY
INTO PERSONAL
SPACE
Journey

Public Presence of the House—Its ability to welcome in opportunity and value

THE JOURNEY

Fame and Reputation
Your Power and Future
Wealth – Fire Place
Fire

Food – Resources – Water
Supply – Area of Abundance
and Prosperity
Ability to receive
Wood – Plants

Marriage/Relationships
Master Bedroom – Intimate
Space – Protected
Mother

Family and Ancestors
I am part of a Family, Tribe
Wisdom Keepers
Wood – Bright – Forceful

Center

Children and Creative
Energies
Metal – The Circle –
Mirror – The Future

Inner Wisdom
Earth – Internal
Learning about Self

TRANSITION
ENTRY AREA

Helpful People
Ability to give
Heaven – Spiritual
Travel (realm to realm)
Transformation

FRONT DOOR – ENTRY
INTO PERSONAL
SPACE
Journey

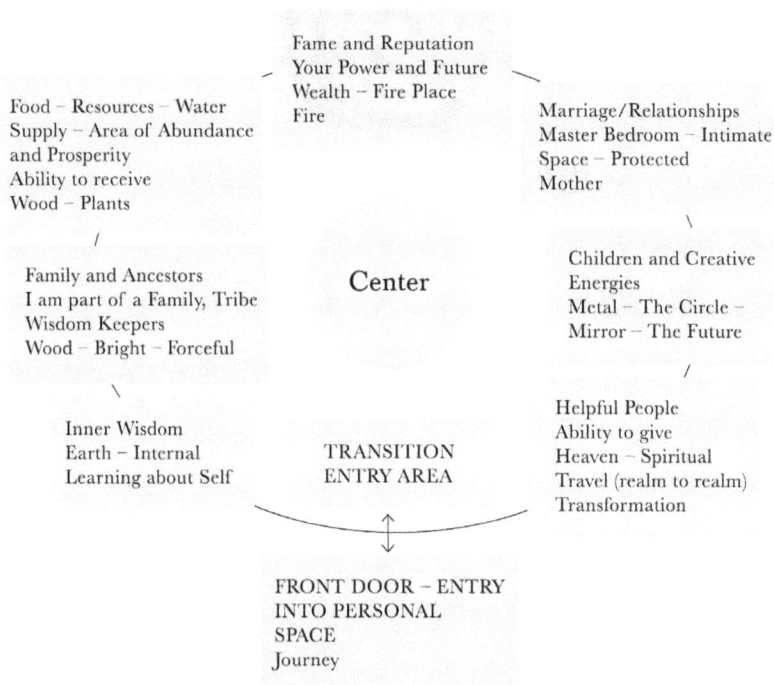

Our main entry door is the beginning of our journey of birth into this lifetime. The journey spirals around in a clockwise motion as we move into an area relating to our discovery into self. As infants we are here now on Earth and learning "who we are" as a human being. Our next step is our connection to our family and tribe— we create connections, identity, and huge growth. As we mature into young adults, we have entered a time of accessing resources and receiving abundance and flow. We reach our pinnacle of power as we move up to the top into the area of fire; our gifts are seen in the world. From the height of self-expression, we move into connecting with another through intimate relationships. A natural energy of male/female that allows life to sustain. After intimate connection, we birth children and/or creative projects that build the future. Finally, we gather all our life's gifts into a place of gathering, spiritual awakening, mentorship, and gratitude to complete life's journey.

Circle of Life—Primal Feng Shui

How do we utilize the circle of life? What does it all mean? The ancient Feng Shui *bagua* and the circle of life symbolize our deep connection to our space. One of the main goals of Feng Shui is to create heaven on Earth for man. Creating a place of balance, harmony and intentional expression will support us on a deep primal level. Every area of our home is vital. Allow your home to support all aspects of your life.

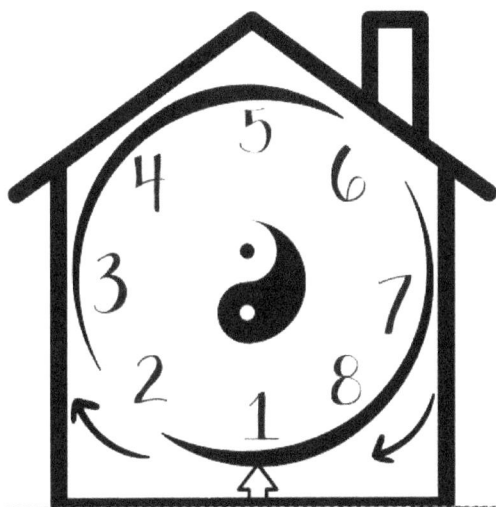

The Circle of Life Sections

1: Here I Am—Birth, Journey of Life, Inhalation
2. I Am a Person—Identify Self as a Human—I Am
3. I Am Heard—Part of a tribe, family, lineage
4. I Grow, I Receive—I shift, change, influence
5. Here I Am—I am Seen—Exhalation, Exaltation, Expression
6. I Expand from 1 to 2—We are—Unity is the seed of life
7 I Create Life—I endow Life, I create the future
8. I Release—I condense, I give
Center—Umbilical Cord—connect to Earth

Here I am
Step 5
Exaltation – Exhalation
My full Expression in the
World – Fire – The Sun
I am seen!

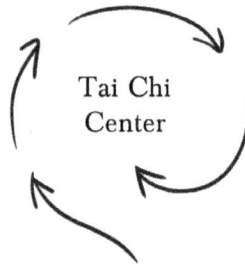

I grow, change, Shift, and
influence life, like the Wind,
Step 4 – Ability to Receive
A young plant growing tall.
I find opportunity – Wood

I expand from 1 to 2 –
Step 6
We are – Unity of Earth –
Male/Female Life's
survival in Marriage

Connect to Family –
Step 3
I am part of a Family,
Tribe
The Past
I am heard,
Thunder – External
Young Plant pops out of
earth

Tai Chi
Center

I create and endow life
– Step 7 – Metal – The
Circle
The Future
The Lake – Internal

Condense & Release –
Step 8
Ability to Give
Heaven – Spiritual
Releasing to ether

Connect to Earth –
Step 2
Identify Self as
Human
I am

Birth
Step 1
Inhalation
Journey of Life
Begins

Our homes are so much more than four walls and a roof. They are true extensions and expressions of our lives.

Man has moved through time from living in a large one room "cave" into homes that contain rooms, each with its own unique purpose and energy. It is essential that our home, our private space is a constant source of nurturing and support.

Edgar Cayce, the Sleeping Prophet states, "The greatest career of any individual is to build the home in such a way and manner as to make it a retreat, as a place where all of those activities are such that it fills the longing that is in the heart and soul of each and every individual."

Everything you need to know about your home is built deep within your core. Go to your gut first, choose what feels safe and secure and uplifting in your home. Your primal wisdom awaits. The home connects to us on our deepest levels. It is of primal importance and when we apply our primal instincts to our home templates, we set the home to pave the way for greater health, peace, stability, and happiness.

NOTES

NOTES

NOTES

NOTES

ABOUT THE AUTHOR

Renae is a certified Feng Shui consultant and teacher with experience in commercial and private properties, community development planning, and business consulting. Her training in Reiki, Rose Alchemy, Pranic Healing, Space Clearing and Japanese martial arts bring a deep understanding of the flow of chi—life force. Renae Jensen is professionally trained and certified with the Feng Shui Institute of America and Instinctive Feng Shui. She is a co-creator of the Conscious Intentional Feng Shui system and Primal Home Feng Shui. She is an active New Jersey real estate agent and specializes in Feng Shui for home sales. Renae has appeared on radio and television programs to share her insight on manifesting through our spaces. She has dedicated her life to promoting healthy spaces through the wisdom of Feng Shui, Space Clearing and Conscious Design. For over twenty years, she has lectured and consulted a wide spectrum of clients and students throughout the United States and Europe.

Renae is former executive marketing director of the International Feng Shui Guild. She was a visionary in the Feng Shui world, and held the first International Feng Shui conferences on the east coast, bringing together masters and wisdom from around the world.

Renae brings her expertise to spaces as small as a child's nursery to urban cities and skyscrapers. The focus is always about creating balanced harmonious healing spaces. Her vision is to foster, guide, educate and uplift people to attain a level of excellence in their lives. Today, as founder of the Conscious Design Institute, Renae has dedicated herself to providing valuable programs to the general public, as well as professionals in the field of real estate, architecture, design, and city planning. Her certification programs follow the Conscious Design path of integrated knowledge, leading us all to a healthier planet, one building at a time.

RenaeJensen@gmail.com
908-797-5225
www.RenaeJensen.com
www.Designharmony.com
www.ConsciousDesignInstitute.com

www.ingramcontent.com/pod-product-compliance
Lightning Source LLC
Chambersburg PA
CBHW031218270326
41931CB00006B/610